# This Is Asperger Syndrome

Written by
Elisa Gagnon
Brenda Smith Myles

Illustrated by
Sachi Tahara

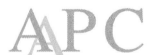

AAPC

Autism Asperger Publishing Co.
P.O. Box 23173
Shawnee Mission, Kansas 66283-0173

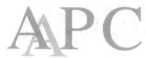

© 1999 by Autism Asperger Publishing Co.
Reprinted 2004
P.O. Box 23173
Shawnee Mission, Kansas 66283-0173

**Publisher's Cataloging-in-Publication**
**(Provided by Quality Books, Inc.)**

Gagnon, Elisa
    This Is Asperger Syndrome / written by Elisa
Gagnon, Brenda Smith Myles ; illustrated by Sachi
Tahara. -- 1st ed.
    p. cm.
    SUMMARY: Introduces children to the world of
their peers who display the confusing behaviors of
Asperger Syndrome.
    Library of Congress Catalog Card Number: 99-73517
    ISBN: 0-9672514-1-9

1. Asperger Syndrome--Juvenile literature.
I. Myles, Brenda.  II. Tahara, Sachi.  III.
Title

RC553.A88M97 1999          616.89'82
          QBI99-1032

Managing Editor: Kirsten McBride
Cover Design: Taku Hagiwara
Production Assistant: Ginny Biddulph
Interior Design/Production: Taku Hagiwara

Printed in the United States of America

## Foreword

***This Is Asperger Syndrome helps you navigate uncharted waters...***

My ten-year-old son, Shawn, has Asperger Syndrome. He has always been fully included in regular education classrooms, but this year he is attending a brand new parochial school. His paraprofessional and I have worked very hard to educate his classmates about Shawn's "invisible disability." They have responded very well, making my son's fourth-grade classroom a welcoming, comfortable place for him. He still must work very hard to navigate the social situations that arise each day, but at least his classmates have appeared to be supportive of his efforts so far.

Educating Shawn's classmates about Asperger Syndrome often makes me feel like I'm venturing into uncharted waters. There is no physical "wheel chair ramp" that can provide my son access to the social world of neurotypical humanity. His ramp can only be constructed out of the attitudes and empathy of the persons with whom he interacts. In addition to exploring uncharted waters and constructing ramps without a permit, I sometimes feel I am walking a tightrope trying to educate his classmates in the hope of shaping their attitudes and their capacity for empathy without making too big a deal out of Shawn's disability.

One of my ventures on the high wire involved sharing Elisa Gagnon and Brenda Smith Myles' book, *This Is Asperger Syndrome,* with my son's classmates. As I read each page, I asked the children to share their reactions by filling in a questionnaire I had written. The questionnaire asked them to compare and contrast the behaviors of the child in the book with the behaviors they had seen in Shawn. Shawn had okayed the questionnaire and thought it would be interesting. I was hoping it would provide me with feedback on how our "ramp construction" was going.

As I started to read the book aloud in his classroom, Shawn asked his paraprofessional to take him out of the room for sensory integration exercises. My heart sunk. Had I embarrassed him? Had I had gone too far? Was *I* perseverating on *his* autism? I continued with the book, too embarrassed to admit that I just might have been adding to my son's difficulties. I comforted myself with the realization that Shawn's classmates were eagerly filling in their questionnaires and asking very thoughtful questions about the character in the book, who faces an entire school of teachers, peers, and even a substitute teacher, who do not understand his disability and rarely give the poor kid a break. I was amazed at how interested the kids were in the book, but I was also worried that perhaps I had botched things up for my son.

A few days later, Shawn's paraprofessional stopped me when I came to pick him up from school. She said that something had happened that I should know about. I always hold my breath when she says that.

It seems that the kids had had a substitute music teacher that day. As Shawn's class were settling into the music room (music is Shawn's most successful class, behavior-wise), Shawn was startled by the realization that he had to go to the bathroom. He jumped out of his seat, his loud voice announcing with unintended bravado, "I gotta use the can!!" The poor substitute teacher was trying to begin the class with the air of confident control that is the hallmark of successful substitute teaching. She had been told a little about Shawn, but felt it was necessary to squelch his behavior, which seemed very much like an offensive move by a class clown. As a result, she countered with a sharp reprimand that began something like, "What do you think you're doing, young man?," and ended by insisting that he rephrase the outburst into the form of a respectful request. She did not know that pouncing upon the behavior of an already startled Shawn usually eliminates the possibility of his learning an important lesson at that given moment.

What Shawn probably experienced at that moment was a feeling that he had just been sucker punched by the substitute music teacher, right on the heels of having been mercilessly ambushed by a sudden need to pee. Finally, after the poor substitute teacher had saved face, Shawn was allowed to escape to the boys' room, not knowing that something truly amazing was about to occur back the music classroom.

At this point the paraprofessional, who was relaying the music class incident to me, paused, peeking up beneath the hand that I was holding across my painfully winced forehead. I was wondering if I had embarrassed my son in front of his classmates to the point that his behavior was regressing. For some reason the paraprofessional was smiling, no, not just smiling–she was beaming. I had yet to hear what had occurred in the music class while Shawn was in the bathroom. The substitute music teacher had relayed to the paraprofessional that immediately after Shawn had left for the bathroom, the children's hands had shot up. They all wanted to inform the substitute that Shawn hadn't meant to be disrespectful. "Don't you know he has Asperger Syndrome?" was the chorus ringing through the music room that day. My son's classmates had then taken turns trying to educate the substitute on what Asperger Syndrome is all about. They were standing up for my son!

When you read *This Is Asperger Syndrome*, you will see exactly which of its pages inspired my son's fourth-grade classmates. As nervous as it makes me to venture into these uncharted waters and to attempt my high wire act, it is moments like this that make it all worthwhile. Thank you, Elisa and Brenda, for touching the hearts of Shawn's classmates. I need all the help I can get with ramp construction.

By the way, the other equally important aspects of my son's ramp are his own feelings of confidence and self-worth. When I finally summoned the courage to inquire about my reading the book in his class, he told me that the book and the questionnaire were a little embarrassing, but not too bad. He had asked to leave the room that day because he had really, *really* needed some sensory integration activities.

*–Jeanne Lyons*, Shawn's mother

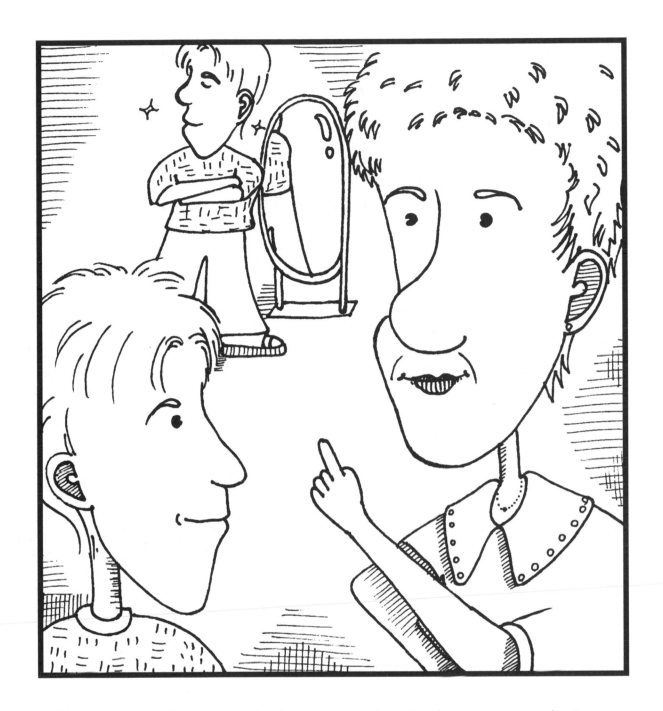

I like to wear the same clothes every day, both summer and winter -- tan pants, an aqua-colored T-shirt, white socks and sandals. Kids at school say I'm strange. Mom says I'm eccentric.
*This is Asperger Syndrome.*

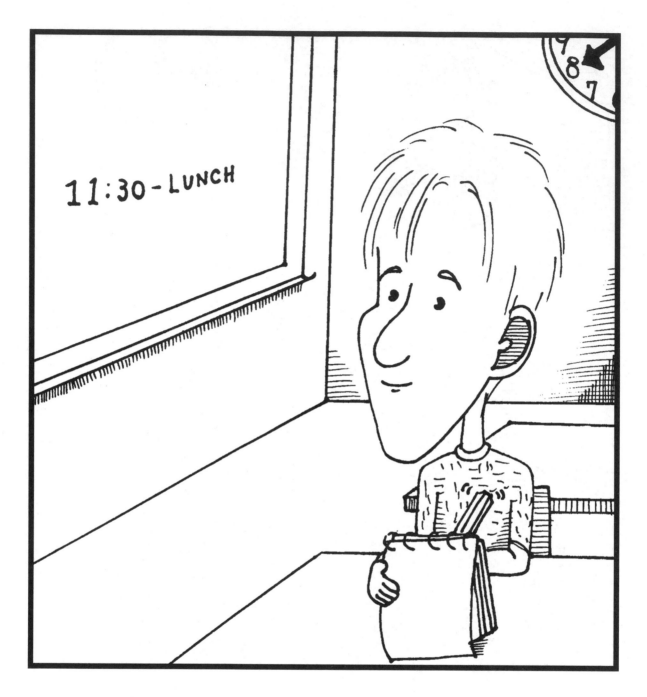

I usually begin my school day by copying the daily schedule from the chalkboard. I carry the schedule in my pocket so I can refer to it when I need to. Most of the time the days at school are the same, but sometimes we have an all-school assembly or an early dismissal. I don't mind as long as I know what is going on, and my schedule helps keep me on track.

*This is Asperger Syndrome.*

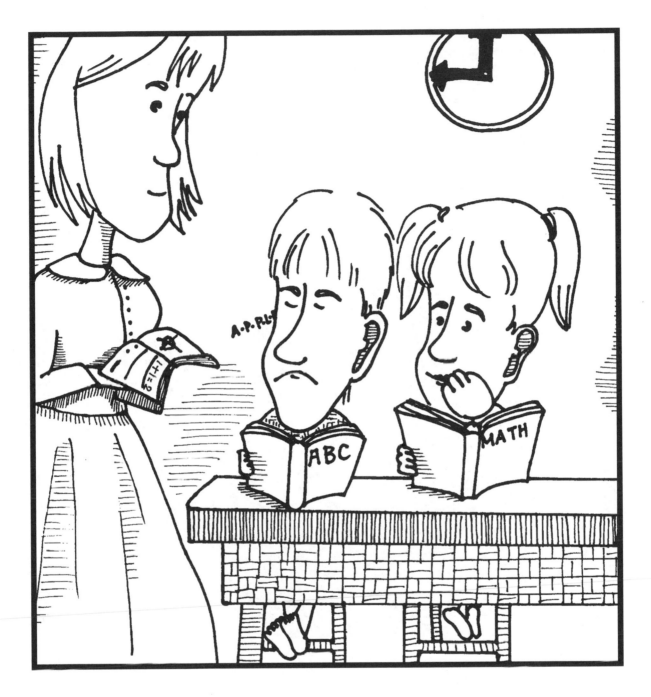

We have a substitute teacher today. I hate substitutes because they never know what to do. At 9:00 o'clock she told us to get out our math books. Everyone knows that 9:00 o'clock is spelling time so I refused to get out my math book.
*This is Asperger Syndrome.*

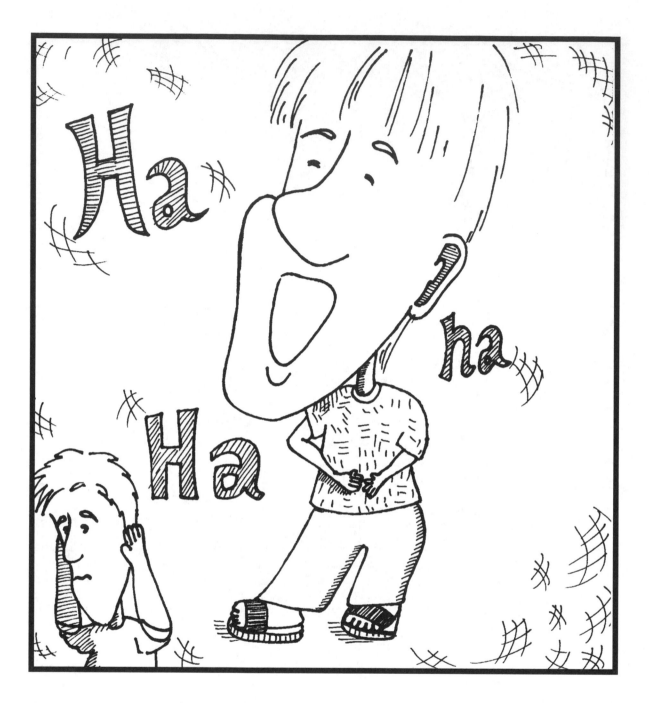

It seems to me that people are always laughing for no reason.
People laugh while watching TV, at the movie theater, at school,
and in restaurants. I try to laugh when other people laugh but the
kids at school say, "Shut up, you laugh too loud."
*This is Asperger Syndrome.*

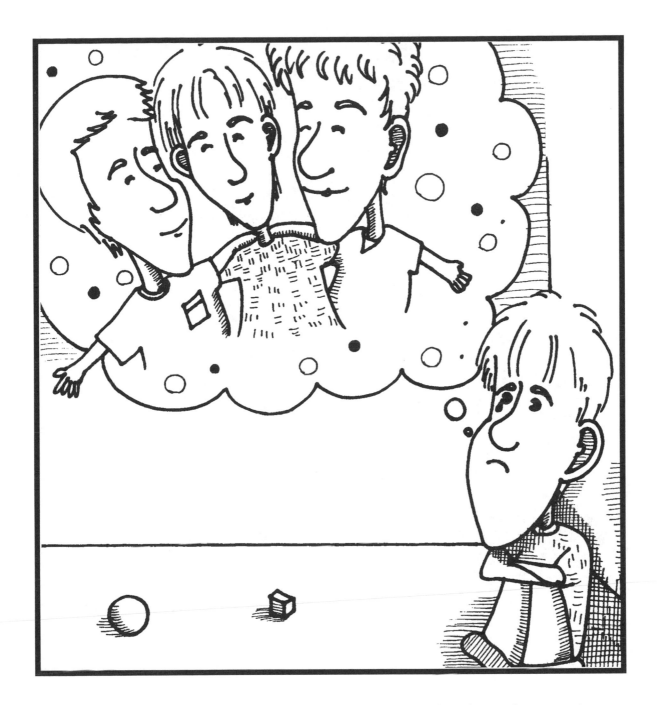

I'm always alone--recess, lunch time, after school. Dad says I'm a loner. Even when there are lots of people around, I still feel alone. I want to have friends but I don't know how.
*This is Asperger Syndrome.*

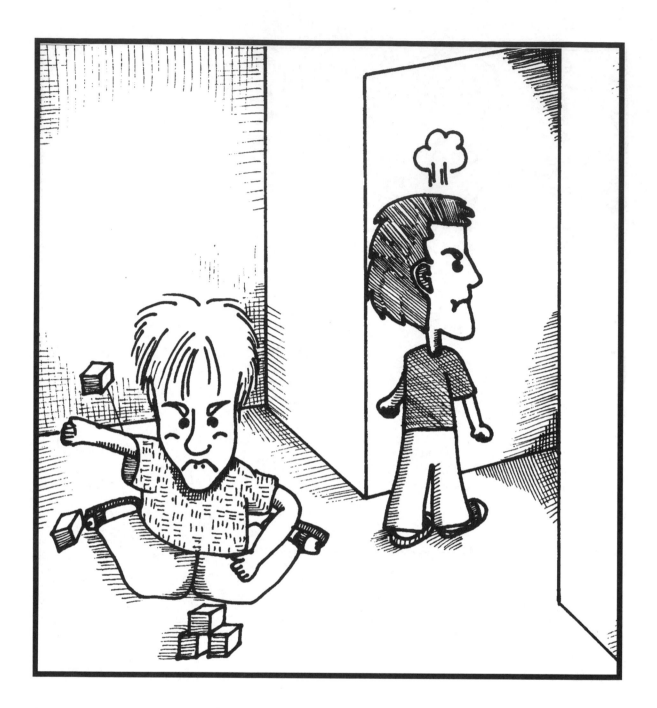

I sometimes try to play with other kids but get upset when they don't play by the rules. They laugh at me or run away. Sometimes this makes me so mad that I hit or kick them.
*This is Asperger Syndrome.*

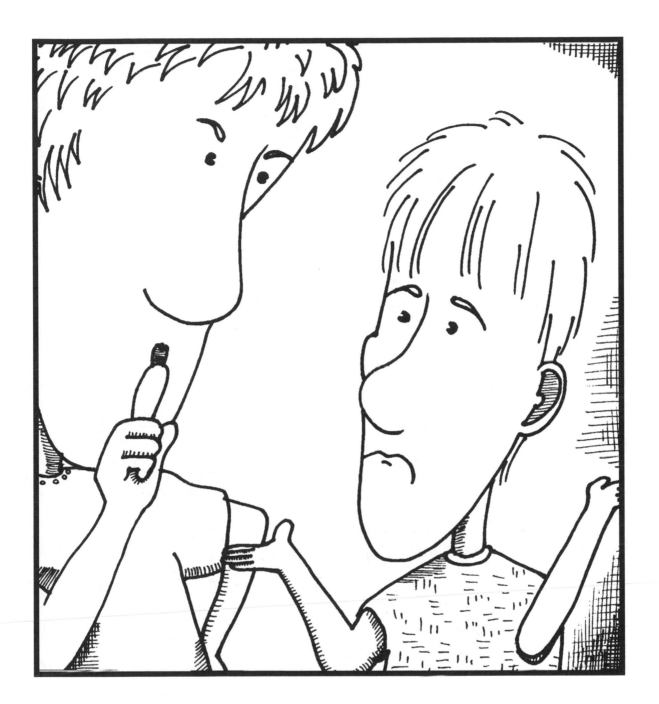

My teacher says I'm rude. I think I'm honest. I don't understand why I can't tell someone that they have bad breath, ugly hair, or to go away because I'm busy.
*This is Asperger Syndrome.*

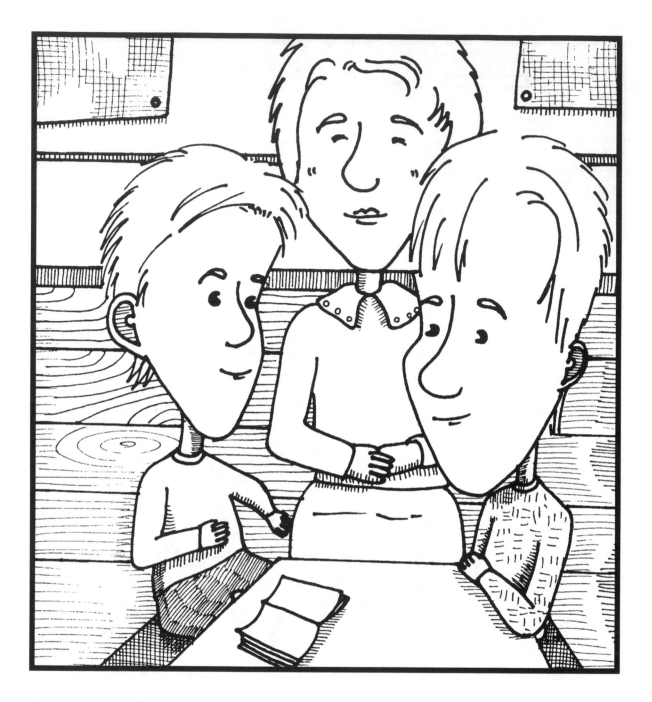

Twice a week I go to social skills training with some of the other students. I work on getting along with people and some of the kids work on being more patient. We are all learning how to listen to our friends when they talk and how to treat other people the way we want to be treated.

*This is Asperger Syndrome.*

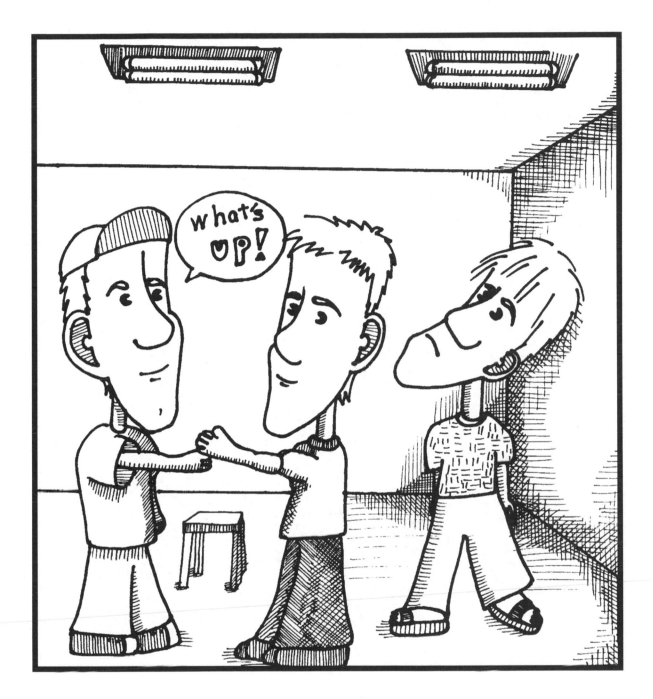

When I walk into the lunch room the kids always say "What's up!" so I look up. I have a great sense of humor but people seldom get my jokes.
*This is Asperger Syndrome.*

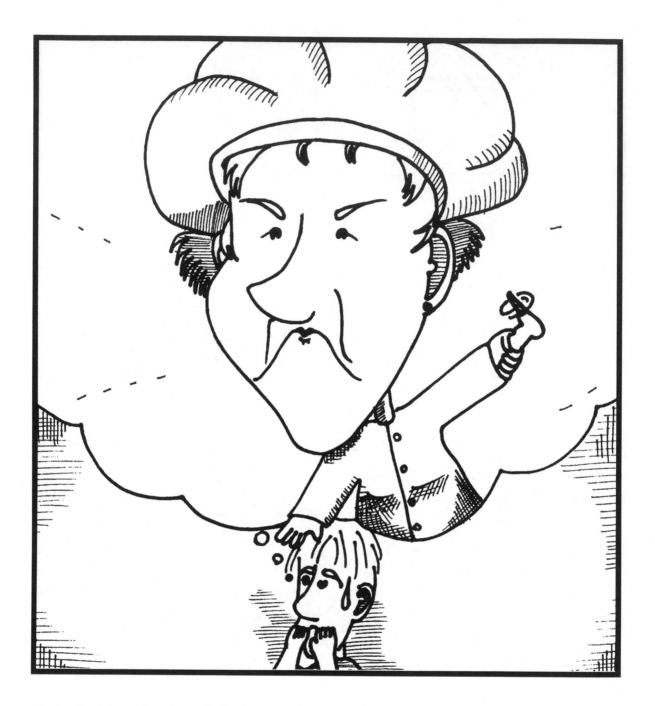

I don't like the lunch lady. Today I asked her for more ice cream. She replied, "You need more ice cream about as much as you need a hole in your head." I got really scared because I thought she wanted to put a hole in my head with a drill.
*This is Asperger Syndrome.*

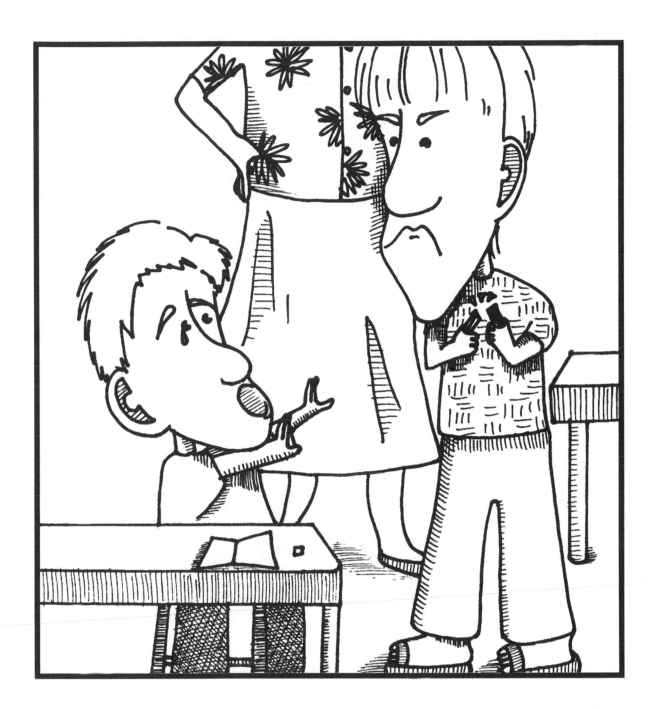

After lunch today, I had trouble concentrating because this kid kept tapping his pencil. I told him to stop but he just looked at me and kept tapping. He continued to tap his pencil even after the teacher told him to stop. When I couldn't stand the noise another second, I grabbed his pencil and broke it. It isn't fair that I'm the one in trouble now.

*This is Asperger Syndrome.*

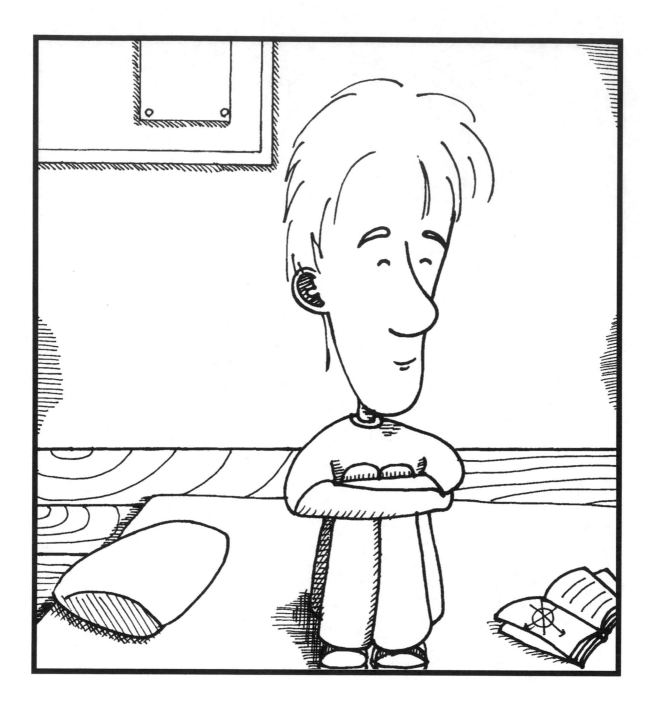

After I broke the pencil, I went to see the school counselor because I felt bad. She had a great idea! The next time a noise is driving me crazy, I will ask to leave the room and go to my safe place. I have special permission to sit there until I am ready to rejoin the class.

*This is Asperger Syndrome.*

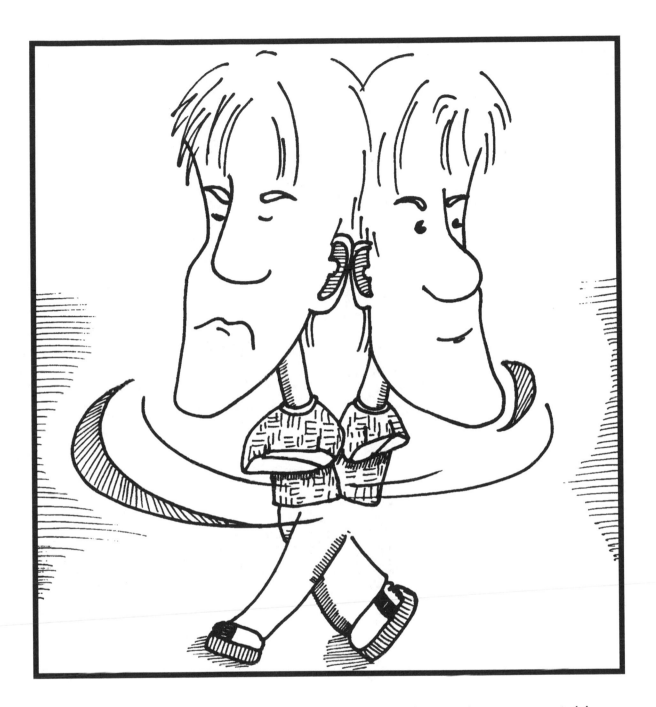

Sometimes when I am angry I can feel my heart beating quickly and I pace back and forth. Sometimes I yell. I don't understand why things have to change all the time.
*This is Asperger Syndrome.*

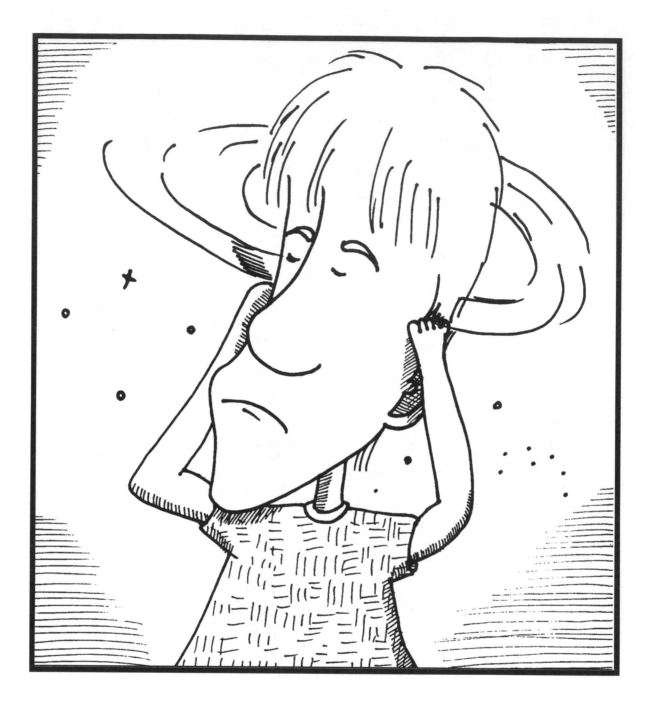

My mind races a hundred miles an hour. My mouth can't keep up with all the thoughts in my head. In the middle of talking about the weather, I suddenly start talking about the space shuttle. My mother tells me to slow down because I'm rambling. Kids at school just quit listening and walk away.
*This is Asperger Syndrome.*

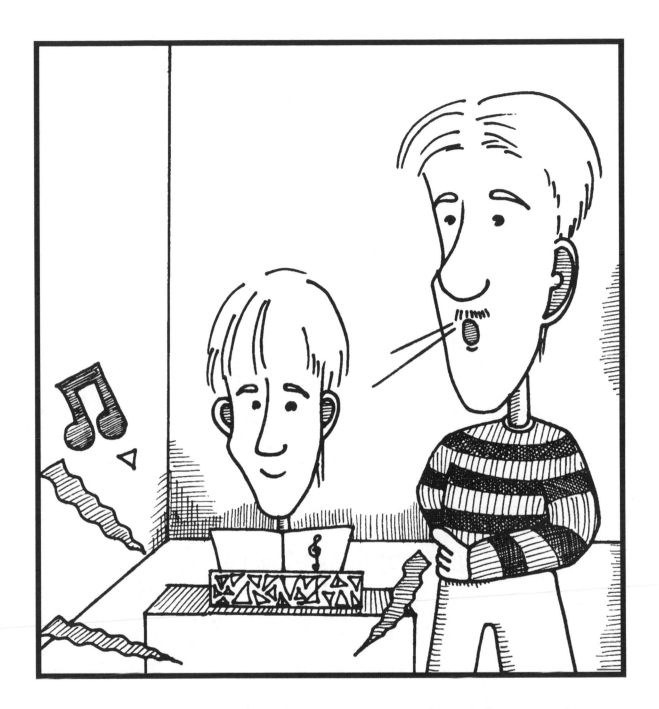

After school I like to play the piano. My Dad said, "Can you bang those keys a little harder?" so I did. I was in big trouble but I'm not sure why.
*This is Asperger Syndrome.*

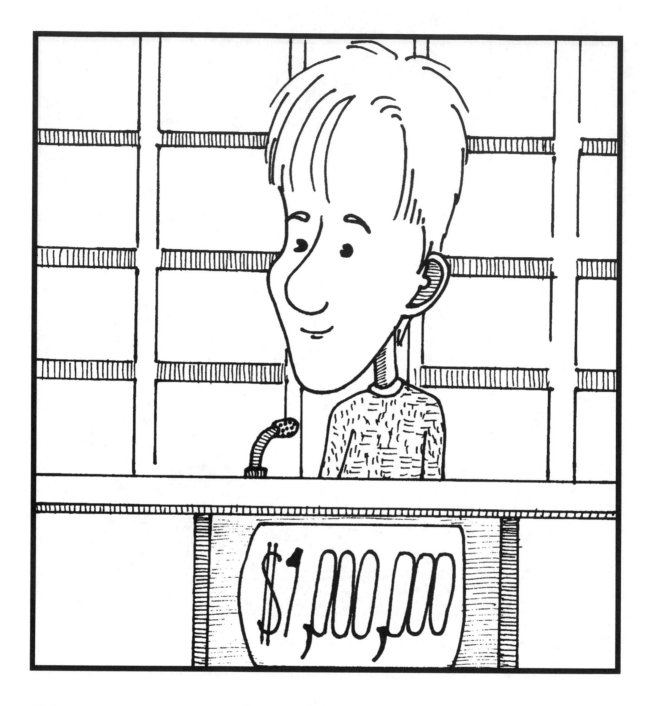

I have a great memory for numbers and facts. When Mom forgets a phone number, she asks me what it is and I always seem to remember. I know I could win lots of money on *Jeopardy* or *Who Wants to Be a Millionaire?*
*This is Asperger Syndrome.*

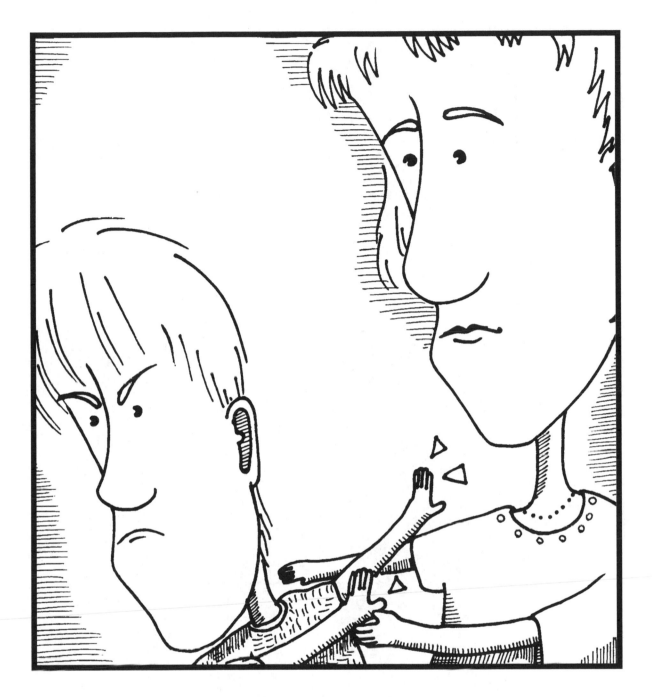

My Aunt Helen came over this afternoon. She is always hugging me. I try to stay away from her because she squeezes too hard and smells like coffee. Last week I told her to leave me alone and when she didn't, I elbowed her right in the stomach. Mom says I hurt Aunt Helen's feelings but I don't care as long as she stops touching me.
*This is Asperger Syndrome.*

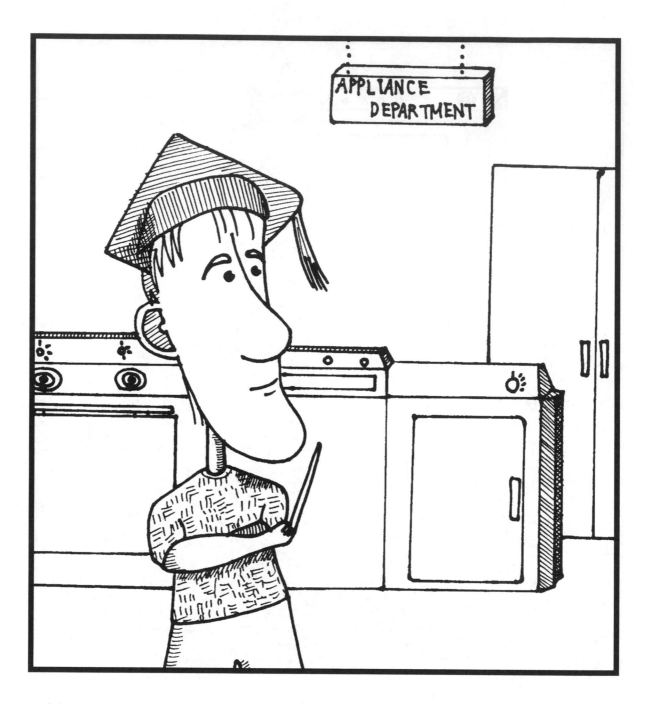

I like to visit the appliance department. Washers and dryers are my favorite and I think I know more about them than any kid in the world. I also check out the appliances in every house I visit, and I love to talk about appliances. It's a fascinating topic but no one ever wants to listen to me talk about them for very long. I don't understand why everyone isn't interested in appliances.
*This is Asperger Syndrome.*

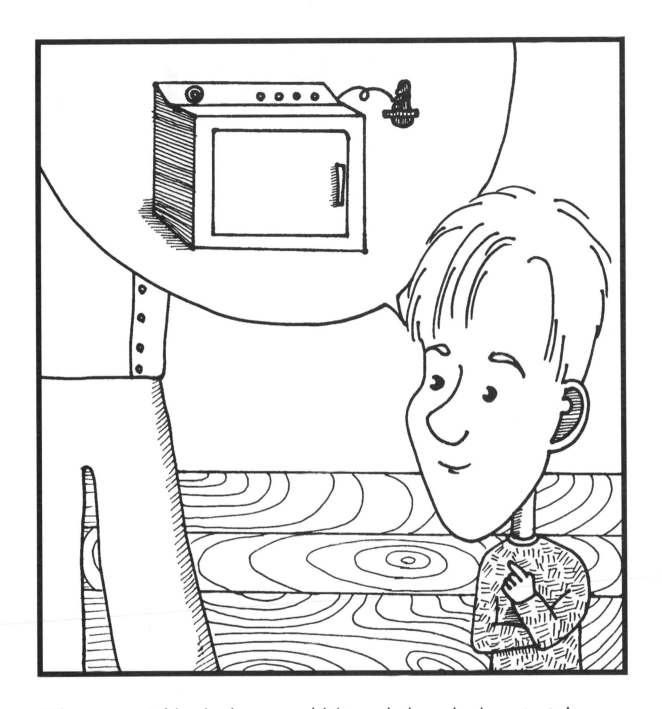

When my neighbor's dryer wouldn't work, he asked me to take a look at it. He was so impressed when I told him exactly what part he needed in order to fix it. It just took a few minutes to fix it once we had the part, and now it works as good as new.
*This is Asperger Syndrome.*

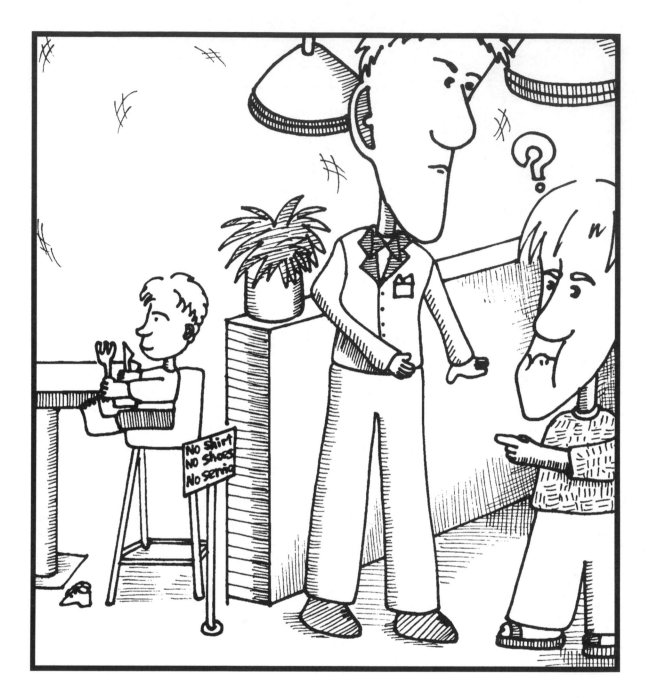

We went out to dinner the other night. When we walked into the restaurant, the first thing I saw was a sign that said "No Shirt, No Shoes, No Service," so I was glad I was wearing shoes and a shirt. There was a barefoot kid next to us eating in a high chair. I told my family and the waitress that the kid needed to wear shoes. When they didn't do anything about it, I yelled for the manager. I was furious when he laughed at me, so I yelled louder. We were finally asked to leave the restaurant. It wasn't fair because we all had on shoes and shirts.
*This is Asperger Syndrome.*

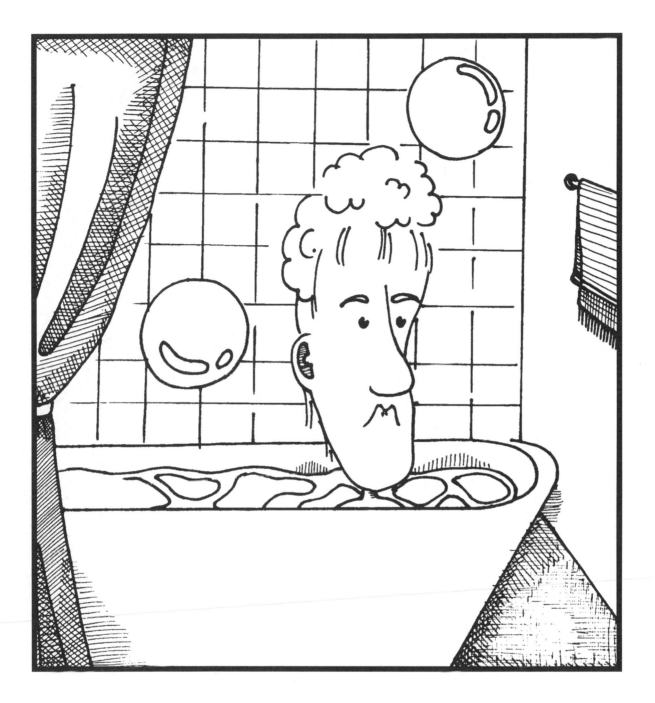

Why do I have to bathe and brush my teeth every day? I hate being wet and I hate the taste of toothpaste. Mom says, "Quit complaining and just do it!" It's easy for her to say because she likes baths and toothpaste.

*This is Asperger Syndrome.*

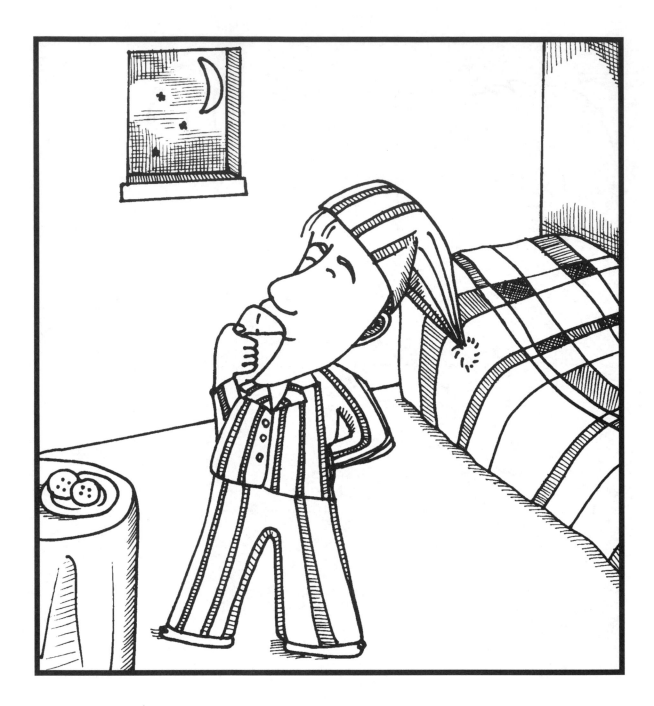

It's finally time for bed. I always eat two cookies and drink one cup of milk at bed time. Before I go to bed, I clear everything out of my room and make sure that there are no wrinkles in the covers. Maybe tomorrow won't be so confusing.
*This is Asperger Syndrome.*

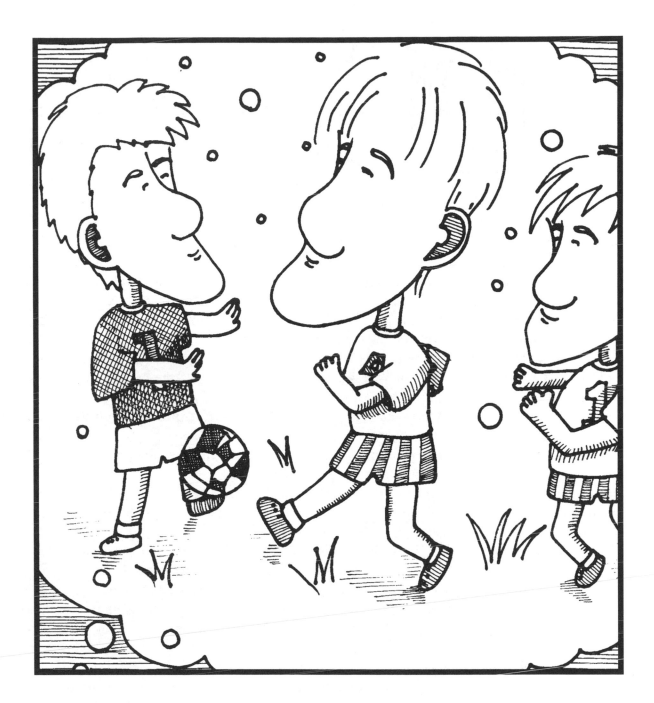

What about tomorrow? I know many things and I want to share what I know with other people. Sometimes I look at things a little differently, but once we find things we have in common we can get along and become good friends.

*This is Asperger Syndrome.*

**Notes on Asperger Syndrome**

Everyone is special. Each of us does certain things well while there are other things that we are not so good at doing. People with Asperger Syndrome (AS) are no different. They bring with them special gifts and challenges. The goal of this book is to help children and youth with AS, as well as their siblings and peers to gain a better understanding of Asperger Syndrome.

Although each person with AS is unique, they often share certain characteristics. For example, individuals with AS often:

1.  Have average to above-average intelligence.
2.  Prefer predictability in their environment. They rely on visual schedules and routines to help them throughout the day. If their routine is changed, they may have difficulty adjusting. People with AS like rules when they understand them. As a result, when rules are broken by others, they may try to stress the importance of following rules or try to prompt a rule-breaker to follow the rule, sometimes in inappropriate ways.
3.  Experience sensory differences. For example, they may like the feel of certain material, and insist on wearing only clothes made out of that material. In addition, people with AS may not like being touched by others. It is often difficult for people with AS to tell others about their sensory needs.
4.  Have voices or speech patterns that are different from those of their peers. Many people have unique voices or speech patterns.
5.  Find it difficult to understand the world around them. They often interpret their environment literally and may have difficulty understanding jokes or idioms. They often have a great sense of humor themselves, however.
6.  Want to have friends, but they often do not know how to make friends easily. They may spend time alone because they have not learned how to have friends. Often, they do not understand the rules of friendships and other social activities.
7.  Share their thoughts openly. They are not rude; they just say what is on their mind. People with AS often say out loud the things that other people only think for fear of offending or hurting others.
8.  Demonstrate strong areas of interest or obsession. For example, a child may be an expert on dinosaurs or know everything about astronomy. They often want to share their information with others, but have difficulty knowing if others are interested in what they have to say.

These are only some of the unique characteristics of AS. There are many others. What characteristics do the people you know have? Remember, everyone is special and if we understand the needs of all people, we can all get along.